# The Sugar Detox Diet

By

Hathai Ross

# The Sugar Detox Diet

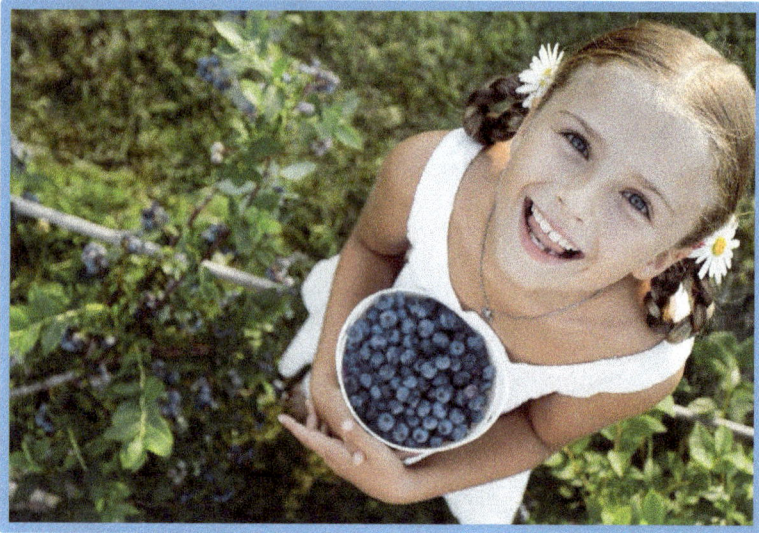

## A Complete Guide with Recipes

Free Yourself from Sugar Addiction and Food Cravings by
Engaging in a 30-Day Whole Food Detox

# Copyright Page

# Forward

The sugar detox is a life-changing process that can help you to get rid of your sugar cravings once and for all. In addition to freeing you from food cravings, this detox will help you to cleanse your body, jumpstart your weight loss plans and set you on the path to a healthier you!

# Acknowledgements

I would like to thank my friends and family for being such willing test subjects throughout my research and writing process. I would also like to thank my husband in particular for his support throughout this exciting journey.

# Table of Contents

# Chapter One: Introduction

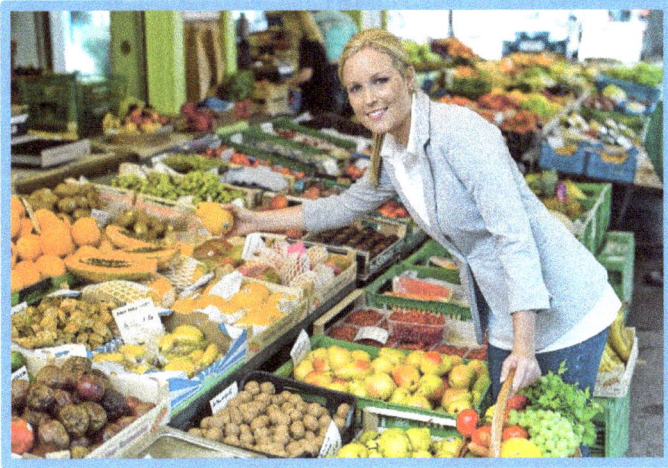

If you read the cover of your favorite health and fitness magazine, you are likely to see headlines with words and phrases like "lose weight fast" and "drop 10 pounds." These claims can be very exciting, but they can also be very misleading. Unfortunately, many people do not understand that losing weight and improving your health is a long-term goal, not a short-term goal. It took you time to gain the extra weight you're carrying so it only makes sense that it will take a little bit of time for you to lose it.

Whether you need to lose weight or not, the chances are good that your health could use some improvement. The modern Western diet seems to be based on high-calorie processed foods loaded with sugar and fat. In fact, you could be addicted to sugar without even knowing it, simply because it is so prevalent in the foods you eat! Over time, the more sugar and processed foods you consume, the more it will have an impact on your body and your health. Before you know it, your body will become toxic and it will not function as well as it once did.

This is where the sugar detox comes in. If you find yourself craving sweets, reaching for that extra cookie or cupcake when you know you don't need it, a sugar detox may be just what you need. Even if you do not struggle with sweet cravings as often as others, you can still benefit from this wonderful detox. A sugar detox is designed to help you lose weight, cut cravings and improve your health by ridding your diet of sugary, high-calorie foods. It could be the dieting solution you have been waiting for.

In this book you will find all the information you need to learn what a detox is, how to plan one and tips for getting through it. Your success in completing a sugar detox depends not only on your commitment to the process but also in how well you plan it – you need to have a wide variety of recipes on hand as well as the ingredients and equipment needed to make them. This book provides all the sugar detox recipes you need including smoothies, juices, breakfasts, soups, salads, entrees, desserts and more. You certainly won't go hungry on your sugar detox!

**So what are you waiting for? Turn the page and start your own sugar detox today!**

# Chapter Two: Understanding the Sugar Detox

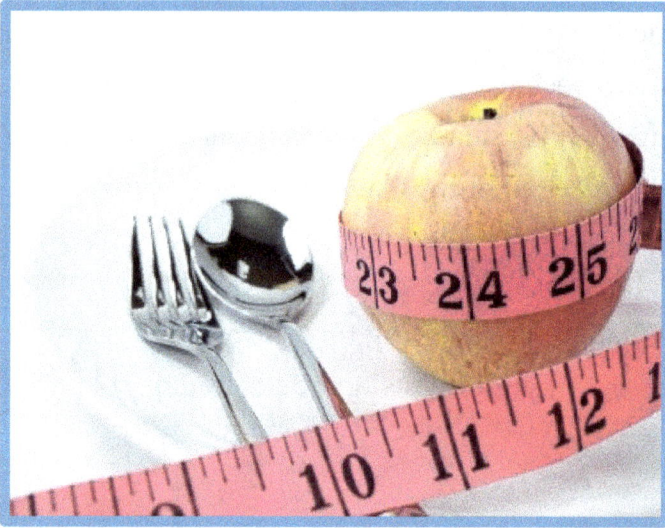

You probably already have a basic understanding of what the sugar detox is and how it can help you – but you should know more than just a few details before you actually start to engage in the detox. Engaging in a detox is a process that shouldn't be entered into lightly. You need to prepare both your body and your mind before you accept the challenge if you truly want to be successful. In this chapter you will learn all of the important details about the sugar detox including what a detox is, how it can benefit you and what foods you should eat and avoid while detoxing.

## 1.) What is a Detox?

The word "detox" is short for "detoxification" and it is typically used to describe a period of clean eating designed to cleanse the body of accumulated wastes and toxins. Your body has many natural detoxification systems in place but, depending on the number of toxins you put into your body on a regular basis, extra toxins may build up. Accumulated toxins can interfere with your body's natural detoxification system which may lead to a number of problems including lethargy, gastrointestinal problems and weight gain.

Before you can fully understand what a detox is and how it works, you need to understand how toxins get into your body in the first place. You may be surprised at all the ways that your body comes into contact with toxins – from the air you breathe to the products you use on your skin and even the food you eat. Commercially raised meats, processed foods, even fruits and vegetables can contain toxins in the form of pesticides, mold and dangerous chemicals. Pollutants in the air may enter the body through your lungs and commercial beauty products can introduce toxins through the skin.

## a.) Types of Detox

Just as there are many reasons why you might engage in a detox, there are different types of detoxes to choose from. In some cases, detoxes are classified by the type of organ they target for detoxification. The body's natural detoxification system involves several of the body's largest organs including the lungs, skin, kidneys, colon and liver. <u>Below you will find a brief overview of each of these types of organ detox</u>:

## Liver

The liver is often identified as the most important detoxification organ in the body – it is responsible for the breakdown of toxins and medications. Once the toxins have been processed, they are excreted from the body through bile and urine. A liver detox requires the intake of plenty of antioxidants as well as vitamins and minerals like vitamin C, selenium, carotene and vitamin E. Consuming amino acids from cruciferous vegetables have also been shown to aid in liver detoxification.

## Kidney

The kidneys are responsible for filtering your blood, removing toxins and diverting them to the urinary system to be flushed from the body. Your kidneys also help to maintain sodium levels in the body – sodium plays an essential role in controlling the build-up of toxins. Drinking plenty of water is the key to detoxing your kidneys because water helps to flush the toxins that your kidneys filter out. Eating fresh fruits and vegetables may also be beneficial because the increased fiber content helps aid digestion.

## Lungs

The lungs are responsible for removing toxins that enter your body through the air you breathe. This is incredibly important because the lungs oxygenate your blood before transporting it throughout your body to your organs. If you breathe in too many toxins, it could affect the ability of your lungs to oxygenate your blood and it could have an effect on the rest of your organs and tissues. Breathing fresh air is the easiest way to detox your lungs, but moderate exercise and deep breathing exercises may help as well.

## Skin

Not only is the skin the largest organ in your body, it also plays a significant role in detoxing. Accumulated toxins can be stored in skin cells which flake off the body – you can also release toxins through perspiration. On the other hand, you can absorb a lot of toxins through your skin as well in using commercial beauty products. Skin brushing is one easy way to help detoxify the skin – it helps to remove dead skin and to stimulate the lymph system which naturally removes toxins from your body.

## Colon

The colon is the last stop in the digestive process and it plays a very important role in detoxification. When it is healthy, your colon helps to detox the body by breaking down wastes and expelling toxins from the body. Over time and with unhealthy eating, however, the function of the colon can be impaired – constipation and other colon diseases can prevent toxins from properly exiting the body, leading it to become toxic. Fiber is an essential part of a colon cleanse because it helps to pass foods through the colon along with any accumulated toxins.

## 2.) Details of the Sugar Detox

While there are many different kinds of detoxes out there, the sugar detox is designed to help you cut your cravings for sweets, break your addiction to sugar and to improve your overall health and eating habits. This sounds like a lot for one diet to accomplish, but the reality is that improving your eating habits can have a drastic effect on all aspects of your health. Swapping out sugary, carb-loaded and processed foods for whole and natural foods is the key to resetting your body and improving your health.

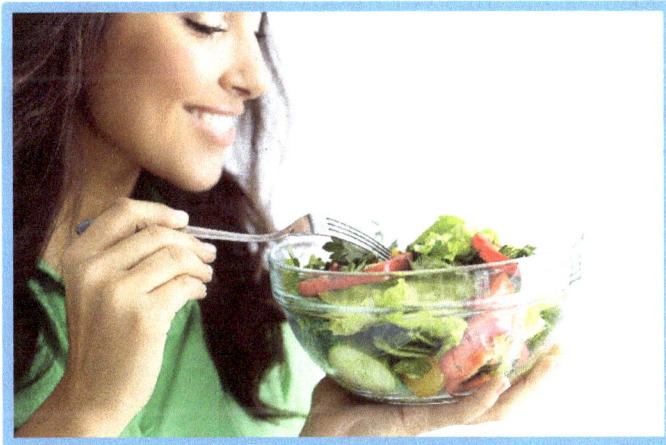

If you perform an online search for a sugar detox, you are likely to find a plethora of results. The detoxes you find will range in regard to their length but, in most cases, a sugar detox should last at least 3 weeks. During the first week or so of your detox your body will begin flushing out stored toxins and absorbing nutrients from the healthy foods you are eating. Over the next two weeks, your body will experience a number of benefits from eating wholesome, natural foods as opposed to processed food.

The goal of a sugar detox is, of course, to change the way your body reacts to sweets. Many people become addicted to sugar without even realizing it – this addiction can take the form of cravings for sweet foods or simply an addiction to the positive feelings your body has after eating something sugary. In eating whole foods, you can change the way your palate reacts to sweets and you can cut down or even eliminate your cravings. Breaking your addiction to sugar will do more than just reduce your cravings, however – it may also help you to lose weight, to improve your energy levels and to increase your concentration.

## 3.) Benefits of the Detox

A detox is often also referred to as a "cleanse," and for good reason. Detoxing your body is similar to the type of spring cleaning you do for your home – it helps you to clean out all of the junk you have sitting around and, when you're finished, you feel like everything is shiny and new. You will feel more energetic with a clarity of mind you have never experienced before. These are just a few of the benefits of a sugar detox, however – <u>below you will find a list of other benefits you can look forward to</u>:

- **Getting rid of excess waste** – you may be carrying around excess waste in your body that is slowing you down. A detox will help to cleanse your body of its toxins, eliminating that extra waste.

- **Strengthening your immune system** – by eating clean, you will be exposing your body to fewer contaminants that could make you sick. Eating whole foods will also cut down on the energy your body expends digesting food, giving it more energy to fight disease.

- **Increasing your energy levels** – accumulated toxins in your body can make you feel sluggish and tired.

Getting rid of those toxins will restore your natural energy and leave you feeling brand new.

- **Improving skin and hair health** – toxins can affect the way you look just as much as they affect the way you feel. Detoxing will help to clear up your skin and will also make your hair shinier.

- **Increasing your mental focus and clarity** – the more you detox your body, the clearer you will be (both physically and mentally). When you are able to focus, you will also find that you become more productive.

- **Reduced symptoms of gastrointestinal upset** – ridding your body of accumulated toxins will help to reduce gas, bloating and lethargy from overeating.

## 4.) Food to Eat and Avoid

The key to detoxing your body and breaking your sugar addiction is to remove sugar and carbs from your diet for at least 3 weeks. The standard sugar detox lasts for 21 days, but you can feel free to extend your detox longer if you like. <u>Below you will find a list of foods you can enjoy freely on your detox as well as a list of foods to avoid</u>:

**Foods to Enjoy Freely:**

| | |
|---|---|
| Fresh vegetables | Ghee (clarified butter) |
| Avocado | Green apple (in moderation) |
| Beans and lentils | Lemon and Lime |
| Beef and lamb | Miracle Noodles |
| Brown rice | Nuts and seeds |
| Chicken and turkey | Olive oil |
| Coconut oil | Quinoa |
| Eggs | Tomatoes |
| Fish and seafood | Under-ripe bananas |
| Fresh herbs and spices | Unsweetened chocolate |

## Foods to Avoid:

Alcohol

Agave nectar

All fruit (except avocado)

All grains (except rice and quinoa)

Artificial sweeteners

Bread and pastries

Candy

Dairy products

All-purpose flour

Honey

Hydrogenated oils

Maple syrup

Oatmeal

Potatoes and yams

Soy

Sugar (all types)

Vinegar

White rice

Yogurt

**Note:** You may be surprised to find that fruit is on the list of foods to avoid – fruit is good for you, after all. But it is important to remember that fruit contains natural sugars and carbs, so it should not be consumed on the sugar detox.

# Chapter Three: Preparing for the Detox

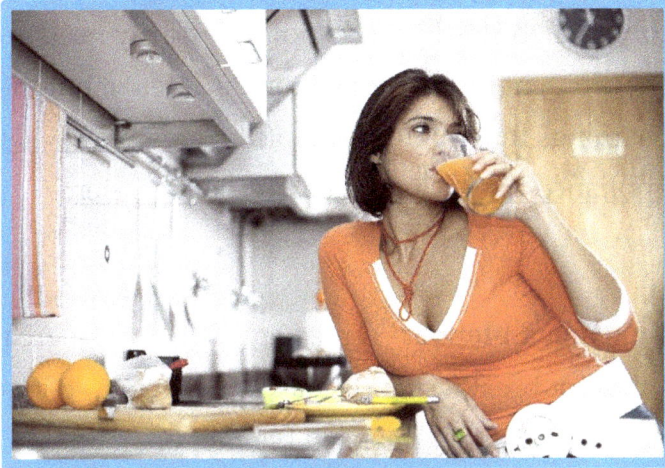

Now that you know the basics about what a sugar detox is and how it can benefit you, you may be ready to move on to the logistics – how do you get started? You already know what foods you can and can't eat on the detox, but there are a few basic preparations you should make. In this chapter you will learn what kind of appliances you will need for the sugar detox and you will receive tips for preparing your kitchen and pantry. You will also receive tips for making the transition into the sugar detox slowly for the maximum benefit.

## 1.) What Equipment Do I Need?

The wonderful thing about a sugar detox is that it is incredibly easy to start! You do not necessarily need any special equipment in order to complete a detox, but there are a few things that might be helpful. <u>Below you will find a list of appliances that will make your detox easier:</u>

- **High-speed blender** – green smoothies are a great option for breakfast and snacks on a detox, so it is very handy to have a high-speed blender on hand.

- **Food processor** – whether you are making your own humus, soup, or snacks a food processor is one appliance you shouldn't be without (you can even use it in place of a blender in many recipes that call for a blender).

- **Cold-press juicer** – juicers can get pretty expensive so don't feel like you absolutely have to go out and buy one. If you are a fan of fresh juice, however, you might find that it is worth the cost to be able to make your own fresh-pressed juices at home during and after your detox.

- **Slow-cooker** – also referred to as a Crock Pot, a slow-cooker is a very convenient cooking method. Slow-cooker recipes typically require little preparation and the food cooks in its own juices which improves flavor and cuts down on the amount of cooking fat you use.

- **Dehydrator** – a dehydrator is a device that removes the moisture from food by heating it at a very low temperature over a long period of time. Again, this is an appliance you do not necessarily need but if you want to experiment with "raw" foods, it will certainly come in handy.

## 2.) Preparing Your Kitchen/Pantry

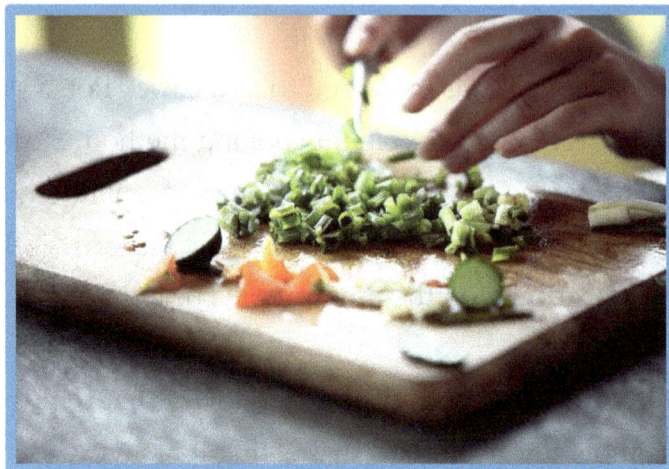

In addition to making sure you have the proper equipment on hand, you also need to stock your kitchen and pantry with detox-friendly foods. Start by cleaning out your pantry and refrigerator, removing any of the foods on the "Foods to Avoid" list. This includes refined sugar, all-purpose flour, frozen dinners, processed snack foods as well as bread and pasta. If you don't intend to come back to these foods after completing the detox, consider donating them to a local food shelter or give it away to family or friends so it does not go to waste.

Once you have made some room in your pantry and refrigerator you can start to stock up on detox-friendly foods. Load your pantry with staples like olive oil, dried beans and lentils, brown rice, nuts and seeds. You can also stock upon dried spices to flavor your dishes. For fresh ingredients, load your refrigerator with fresh herbs and vegetables, lemon and lime for flavoring, tomatoes, and fresh protein like chicken, turkey, beef and lamb.

Because the detox will last for several weeks, you want to pace yourself in stocking your refrigerator with perishable items. Start with enough food for 5 to 7 days and then go shopping again to restock. For the freshest ingredients, check the organic section of your local grocery store or stop in to your local health food store. In the spring and summer months you may even be able to find fresh produce at a local farmers market or by participating in a farm share or community-supported agriculture (CSA) program.

## 3.) Making the Transition

When making any major changes to your dietary habits, it is a good idea to make the transition slowly. You do not want to shock your body by suddenly restricting your diet or reducing your daily calorie intake. To transition into the sugar detox, you might try eliminating one major food from the "Foods to Avoid" list each day over a period of 3 to 5 days. While you do so, try to increase your consumption of the foods on the "Foods to Enjoy Freely" list to compensate. By the time you are ready to start the cleanse, your body will be ready to go.

As you cleanse your body, you should expect a few side effects. Not all of these side effects are going to be unpleasant and they may not even last more than two or three days. Just to be prepared, however, you would be wise to review this list of potential side effects:

- Headaches
- Flu or cold-like symptoms
- Lethargy, loss of energy
- Gas or bloating
- Irritability

- Diarrhea or constipation
- Body odor or bad breath
- Difficulty sleeping

You may also experience some positive side effects, particularly as you get further along in the cleanse:

- Clearer skin
- Reduced food/sugar cravings
- Increased and consistent energy
- Regular bowel movements
- Elevated mood
- Improved sleep patterns
- Weight loss/fat loss
- Increased sense of taste

# Chapter Four: Exercise While Detoxing

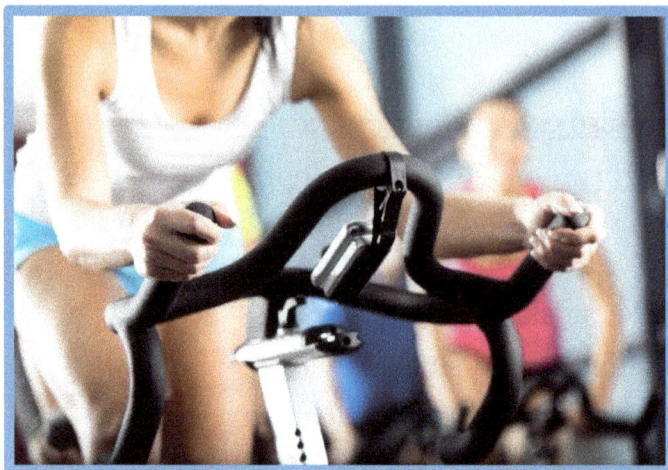

Exercise plays an important role in weight loss and overall health, but it can also be useful in helping you to achieve your detox goals. It is important to remember, however, that you shouldn't participate in vigorous exercise while on a detox until you know how your body is going to handle it. As you will learn in this chapter, however, regular to moderate exercise can help to flush toxins from your body more quickly, revving up the effects of your sugar detox. Keep reading to learn more!

## 1.) How Exercise Benefits a Detox

The key to detoxifying your body is to get your blood pumping and your organs working. Exercise not only increases your heart rate (and thus your blood flow), but it also increases your rate of respiration. The more fresh air you take in, the more oxygen will be delivered to your blood and the better your body will be able to carry out its natural detoxification processes.

As it has been mentioned, moderate exercise is the way to go while participating in the sugar detox. Since you are eating whole foods, your daily calorie intake may be lower than your body is used to so you don't want to overextend yourself with vigorous exercise or training. Mild to moderate exercise helps to activate the lymphatic system, the system that is responsible for filtering and excreting toxins from your body.

## 2.) How to Exercise While Detoxing

When it comes to exercising during a detox, you have many options. One of the best exercises you can do is take a 20-minute walk once a day – this type of moderate exercise is typically the most beneficial while participating in a detox. If you don't have time for a 20-minute walk, try squeezing in two 10-minute walks twice a day. Even if you are only able to get in a walk 3 to 4 times per week, it will still help to benefit your detox.

Yoga has also been said to be very good for detoxifying the body. Twisting poses help to move food along through the digestive system while also compressing the blood vessels around essential organs – this serves to stimulate blood flow, increasing the absorption of nutrients and the removal of toxins. Yoga also encourages deep breathing which increases the oxygenation of your blood and helps your lungs to filter out airborne toxins.

# Chapter Five: Sugar Detox Recipes

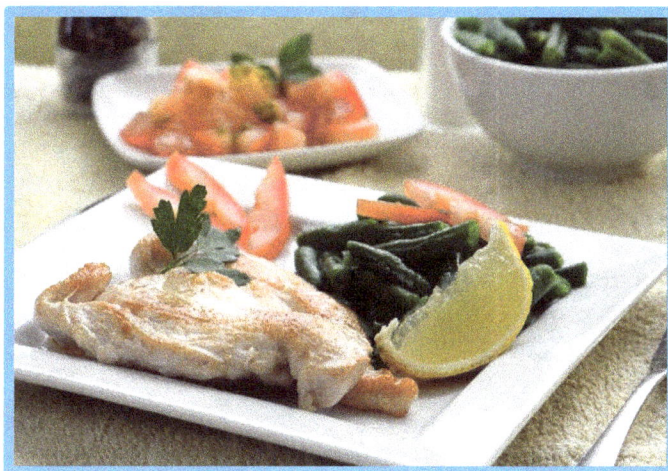

By now you should know everything you need to know before starting the sugar detox. You have received valuable information about what a detox is and how it can benefit you – you've also received tips for getting started and for exercising while on the detox. In this chapter you will receive dozens of delicious recipes to enjoy while following the sugar detox. The key to sticking to the detox is making sure that you don't get bored – with the help of these recipes, you certainly won't have that problem!

## 1.) *Juices and Smoothies*

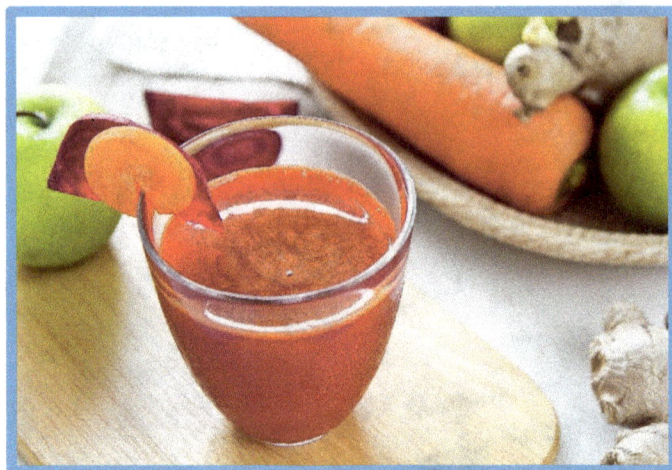

## Recipes Included in this Section:

Super Green Mint Smoothie

Avocado Cucumber Smoothie

Refreshing Cilantro Lime
Smoothie

Broccoli Beet Smoothie

Almond Spinach Smoothie

Spicy Carrot Tomato Juice

Fresh Celery Kale Juice

Simple Salad Greens Juice

Parsley Mint Juice with Lime

Ginger Beet Juice

## Super Green Mint Smoothie

**Servings:** 2

**Prep Time**: 5 minutes

**Ingredients**:

- 2 cups fresh chopped kale
- 2 medium stalks celery, chopped
- ¼ cup fresh parsley
- ¼ cup fresh mint leaves
- 1 cup unsweetened almond milk
- ½ cup ice cubes
- 1 tablespoon fresh lemon juice

**Instructions**:

1. Combine the kale, parsley, mint and almond milk in a blender.
2. Blend until smooth and well combined.
3. Add the remaining ingredients and blend until smooth.
4. Pour into glasses and serve immediately.

## Avocado Cucumber Smoothie

**Servings: 1**

**Prep Time**: 5 minutes

**Ingredients**:

- 1 cup chopped kale leaves
- ½ small seedless cucumber, chopped
- ¼ cup fresh cilantro
- ¼ ripe avocado, peeled and pitted
- ½ cup coconut water, chilled
- ½ inch fresh grated ginger

**Instructions**:

1. Combine the kale, cucumber and cilantro with the coconut water in a blender.
2. Blend until smooth and well combined.
3. Add the remaining ingredients and blend until smooth.
4. Pour into a glass and serve immediately.

## Refreshing Cilantro Lime Smoothie

**Servings:** 2

**Prep Time**: 5 minutes

**Ingredients**:

- 1 bunch fresh cilantro
- 2 medium stalks celery, chopped
- 1 cup chopped romaine lettuce
- ¾ cup unsweetened coconut milk
- 2 tablespoons fresh lime juice
- 1 scoop vegan protein powder

**Instructions**:

1. Combine the cilantro, celery, romaine and coconut milk in a blender.
2. Blend until smooth and well combined.
3. Add the remaining ingredients and blend until smooth.
4. Pour into glasses and serve immediately.

## Broccoli Beet Smoothie

**Servings:** 2

**Prep Time**: 5 minutes

**Ingredients**:

- 1 cup chopped broccoli florets
- 1 small beet, peeled and chopped
- 1 cup chopped kale leaves
- 1 cup unsweetened coconut milk
- 1 tablespoon fresh lemon juice
- ½ inch fresh grated ginger

**Instructions**:

1. Combine the broccoli, beet, kale and coconut milk in a blender.
2. Blend until smooth and well combined.
3. Add the remaining ingredients and blend until smooth.
4. Pour into glasses and serve immediately.

## Almond Spinach Smoothie

**Servings:** 2

**Prep Time**: 5 minutes

**Ingredients**:

- 2 cups fresh baby spinach
- ½ small seedless cucumber, chopped
- ¼ cup fresh parsley
- ¾ cup unsweetened almond milk
- 1 tablespoon fresh lime juice
- 2 tablespoons chopped almonds

**Instructions**:

1. Combine the spinach, cucumber, parsley and almond milk in a blender.
2. Blend until smooth and well combined.
3. Add the remaining ingredients and blend until smooth.
4. Pour into glasses and serve immediately.

## Spicy Carrot Tomato Juice

**Servings:** 2

**Prep Time**: 5 minutes

**Ingredients**:

- 4 large carrots
- 3 medium ripe tomatoes
- 2 small red peppers, cored
- 2 large stalks celery
- 2 cups fresh baby spinach
- 3 cloves garlic, peeled
- 1 jalapeno, seeded

**Instructions**:

1. Rinse all ingredients well and chop them as needed to fit into the juicer.
2. Place a large glass or pitcher under the spout of the juicer.
3. Feed the ingredients through the juicer in the order listed.
4. Stir the juice well and pour into glasses to serve.

## Fresh Celery Kale Juice

**Servings:** 2

**Prep Time**: 5 minutes

**Ingredients**:

- 4 large stalks celery
- 2 large leaves curly kale
- ½ small seedless cucumber
- ½ fresh lemon, peeled

**Instructions**:

1. Rinse all ingredients well and chop them as needed to fit into the juicer.
2. Place a large glass or pitcher under the spout of the juicer.
3. Feed the ingredients through the juicer in the order listed.
4. Stir the juice well and pour into glasses to serve.

## Simple Salad Greens Juice

**Servings:** 2

**Prep Time:** 5 minutes

**Ingredients:**

- 2 large leaves romaine lettuce
- 2 large leaves kale
- 1 cup fresh baby spinach
- 1 handful fresh parsley
- 1 handful fresh cilantro
- 1 inch fresh ginger root

**Instructions:**

1. Rinse all ingredients well and chop them as needed to fit into the juicer.
2. Place a large glass or pitcher under the spout of the juicer.
3. Feed the ingredients through the juicer in the order listed.
4. Stir the juice well and pour into glasses to serve.

## Parsley Mint Juice with Lime

**Servings:** 2

**Prep Time**: 5 minutes

### Ingredients:

- 1 bunch fresh flat-leaf parsley
- ½ bunch fresh mint leaves
- 2 large stalks celery
- 1 small seedless cucumber
- 1 medium carrot
- 1 small lime, peeled

### Instructions:

1. Rinse all ingredients well and chop them as needed to fit into the juicer.
2. Place a large glass or pitcher under the spout of the juicer.
3. Feed the ingredients through the juicer in the order listed.
4. Stir the juice well and pour into glasses to serve.

## Ginger Beet Juice

**Servings:** 2

**Prep Time:** 5 minutes

**Ingredients:**

- 2 large leaves kale
- 2 medium beets, scrubbed and chopped
- 1 cup fresh beet greens
- 1 large stalk celery
- 1 inch fresh ginger root

**Instructions:**

1. Rinse all ingredients well and chop them as needed to fit into the juicer.
2. Place a large glass or pitcher under the spout of the juicer.
3. Feed the ingredients through the juicer in the order listed.
4. Stir the juice well and pour into glasses to serve.

## *2.) Breakfast Options*

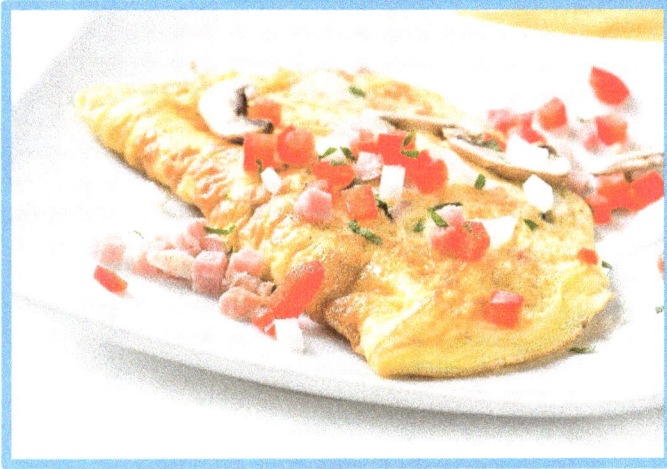

## **Recipes Included in this Section:**

Pumpkin Cinnamon Pancakes

Coconut Flour Pancakes

Carrot Pumpkin Muffins

Almond Flour Muffins

Single-Serve Egg Cups

Tomato Basil Omelet

Mushroom Scallion Omelet

Walnut Breakfast Quinoa

Buckwheat Porridge

Cinnamon Baked Quinoa

## Pumpkin Cinnamon Pancakes

**Servings**: 2

**Prep Time**: 5 minutes

**Cook Time**: 15 minutes

**Ingredients**:

- 4 large eggs
- ½ cup pumpkin puree
- ¾ teaspoon vanilla extract
- 1 teaspoon pumpkin pie spice
- ¼ teaspoon baking soda
- Pinch salt

**Instructions**:

1. Whisk together the eggs, pumpkin and vanilla extract in a bowl.
2. In a separate bowl, stir together the pumpkin pie spice, baking soda and salt.
3. Add the dry ingredients to the wet and whisk smooth.
4. Liberally grease a heavy skillet and heat it over medium heat.

5. Spoon the batter onto the skillet in heaping tablespoons and cook for 1 to 2 minutes until bubbles appear on the surface.
6. Flip the pancakes and cook until browned underneath.
7. Transfer the pancakes to a plate and repeat with the remaining batter.

## Coconut Flour Pancakes

**Servings**: 2

**Prep Time**: 5 minutes

**Cook Time**: 10 minutes

**Ingredients**:

- 1 cup unsweetened coconut milk
- ½ cup coconut flour
- 4 large egg whites
- 1 ½ teaspoons vanilla extract
- 1 teaspoon baking powder
- ½ teaspoon ground cinnamon
- ¼ teaspoon salt

**Instructions**:

1. Combine all of the ingredients in a food processor and blend until smooth.
2. Grease a nonstick skillet and heat it over medium-high heat.
3. Spoon the batter into the skillet in heaping tablespoons and cook for 1 to 2 minutes on each side until golden.

4. Transfer the pancakes to a plate and repeat with the remaining batter.
5. Serve the pancakes warm.

## Carrot Pumpkin Muffins

**Servings**: 12

**Prep Time**: 5 minutes

**Cook Time**: 40 minutes

**Ingredients**:

- 6 large eggs
- ½ cup melted coconut oil
- ¼ cup pumpkin puree
- 1 medium banana, mashed (under-ripe)
- ¾ teaspoon vanilla extract
- ½ cup coconut flour
- 3 teaspoons pumpkin pie spice
- ¼ teaspoon baking soda
- Pinch salt
- 3 cups grated carrot

**Instructions**:

1. Preheat the oven to 350°F and line a regular muffin pan with paper liners.
2. Whisk together the eggs, pumpkin, coconut oil, banana and vanilla extract in a mixing bowl.

3. In a separate bowl, stir together the coconut flour, baking soda, pumpkin pie spice and salt.

4. Add the dry ingredients to the wet and stir until well combined.

5. Fold in the carrots then spoon about ¼ cup of batter into each cup.

6. Bake for 35 to 40 minutes until a knife inserted in the center comes out clean.

7. Cool the muffins in the pan for 5 minutes then turn out onto a wire rack to cool completely.

## Almond Flour Muffins

**Servings**: 12

**Prep Time**: 5 minutes

**Cook Time**: 15 minutes

**Ingredients**:

- 4 cups almond flour
- 8 large eggs
- 2 teaspoons apple cider vinegar
- 1 teaspoon baking soda
- 1 teaspoon ground cinnamon
- Pinch ground nutmeg

**Instructions**:

1. Preheat the oven to 350°F and line a muffin pan with paper liners.
2. Stir together the dry ingredients in a mixing bowl.
3. Beat in the eggs until the batter is well combined.
4. Spoon about ¼ cup of the batter into each cup.
5. Bake for 15 minutes until lightly browned on the edges.
6. Cool for 20 minutes in the pan then serve warm.

## Single-Serve Egg Cups

**Servings**: 12 to 16

**Prep Time**: 5 minutes

**Cook Time**: 10 minutes

**Ingredients**:

- 8 large eggs
- ½ cup unsweetened almond milk
- ½ teaspoon black pepper
- ¼ teaspoon salt
- ½ cup diced ham
- ¼ cup diced mushroom
- ¼ cup diced yellow onion
- 1 tablespoon fresh chopped parsley

**Instructions**:

1. Preheat the oven to 375°F and grease a regular muffin pan.
2. Whisk together the eggs, almond milk, salt and pepper in a mixing bowl.
3. Stir in the chopped vegetables and ham then fill each cup with the egg mixture.

4. Bake for 8 to 10 minutes until the egg is puffed and just set in the middle.

5. Cool for 3 minutes then remove from the pan to serve.

## Tomato Basil Omelet

**Servings**: 1

**Prep Time**: 5 minutes

**Cook Time**: 10 minutes

**Ingredients**:

- 2 teaspoons olive oil
- 2 large eggs
- 1 tablespoon unsweetened almond milk
- Pinch salt and pepper
- 1 small ripe tomato, diced
- 4 fresh basil leaves, chopped

**Instructions**:

1. Heat 1 teaspoon oil in a small skillet over medium heat.
2. Add the tomatoes and basil and cook for 2 to 3 minutes until heated through.
3. Transfer the vegetables to a bowl and set aside.
4. Heat the remaining teaspoon of oil in the skillet over medium-high heat.
5. Whisk together the eggs, coconut milk, salt and pepper in a small bowl.

6.  Pour the egg mixture into the skillet and tilt it to distribute evenly.
7.  Let the egg mixture cook for about 1 minute then scrape down the sides.
8.  Cook for another 2 minutes or so until the egg is almost set.
9.  Spoon the vegetable mixture over half of the omelet and fold the empty half over top.
10. Cook for 30 seconds or so until the egg is set then transfer to a plate to serve.

## Mushroom Scallion Omelet

**Servings**: 1

**Prep Time**: 5 minutes

**Cook Time**: 10 minutes

**Ingredients**:

- 2 teaspoons olive oil
- 2 large eggs
- 1 tablespoon unsweetened coconut milk
- Pinch salt and pepper
- ½ cup diced mushrooms
- 1 medium scallion, sliced

**Instructions**:

1. Heat 1 teaspoon oil in a small skillet over medium heat.
2. Add the mushrooms and scallion and cook for 2 to 3 minutes until heated through.
3. Transfer the vegetables to a bowl and set aside.
4. Heat the remaining teaspoon of oil in the skillet over medium-high heat.
5. Whisk together the eggs, coconut milk, salt and pepper in a small bowl.

6. Pour the egg mixture into the skillet and tilt it to distribute evenly.

7. Let the egg mixture cook for about 1 minute then scrape down the sides.

8. Cook for another 2 minutes or so until the egg is almost set.

9. Spoon the vegetable mixture over half of the omelet and fold the empty half over top.

10. Cook for 30 seconds or so until the egg is set then transfer to a plate to serve.

## Walnut Breakfast Quinoa

**Servings**: 2

**Prep Time**: 5 minutes

**Cook Time**: 20 minutes

**Ingredients**:

- 2 cups unsweetened coconut milk
- 1 cup dry quinoa, rinsed well
- 1/8 teaspoon ground cinnamon
- ¼ cup chopped walnuts

**Instructions**:

1. Place the milk in a small saucepan and bring to a boil.
2. Whisk in the quinoa and return to a boil then reduce heat and simmer for about 15 minutes.
3. Whisk in the cinnamon then cook for about 8 more minutes, covered, until most of the milk has been absorbed.
4. Spoon into bowls and sprinkle with walnuts to serve.

## Buckwheat Porridge

**Servings**: 1

**Prep Time**: 2 minutes

**Cook Time**: 6 minutes

**Ingredients**:

- ¼ cup raw buckwheat groats
- ¼ cup unsweetened almond milk
- 1 cup water
- Pinch ground cinnamon

**Instructions**:

1. Place the groats in a spice grinder and grind well – it is okay if there are some larger pieces left.
2. Whisk together the ground groats with the water and almond milk in a small saucepan.
3. Bring to a boil then reduce heat and simmer for 5 to 6 minutes until thickened.
4. Stir in the ground cinnamon to serve.

## Cinnamon Baked Quinoa

**Servings**: 8 to 10

**Prep Time**: 5 minutes

**Cook Time**: 25 minutes

**Ingredients**:

- 2 ½ cups cooked quinoa
- 4 large eggs
- 1/3 cup unsweetened almond milk
- 3 teaspoons ground cinnamon
- 1 teaspoon vanilla extract

**Instructions**:

1. Preheat the oven to 375°F and line a square baking pan with parchment paper.
2. Whisk together the eggs, almond milk, cinnamon and vanilla extract in a mixing bowl.
3. Stir in the cooked quinoa until just combined then spoon into the baking dish.
4. Bake for 20 to 25 minutes until the top is golden brown.
5. Remove the parchment (along with the baked quinoa) from the pan and cool completely.

6. Cut the quinoa bake into squares to serve.

## 3.) Soups and Salads

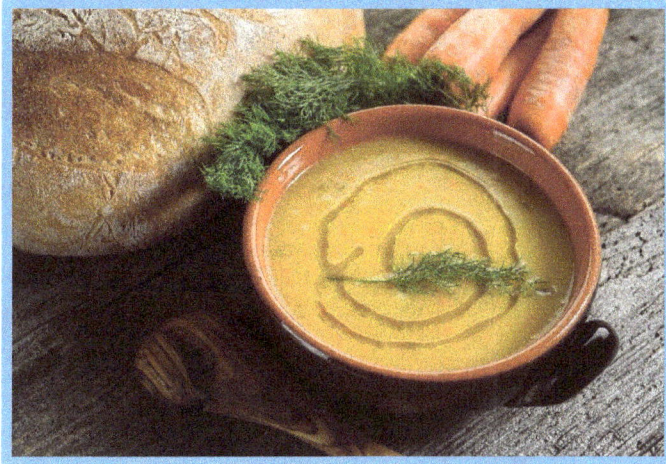

### Recipes Included in this Section:

Cool Cucumber Soup

Creamy Mushroom Bisque

Carrot Ginger Soup

Tomato Gazpacho

Cream of Broccoli Soup

Brussels Sprouts Kale Salad

Colorful Cabbage Slaw

Spinach Basil Lime Salad

Spring Fling Salad

## Cool Cucumber Soup

**Servings**: 6 to 8

**Prep Time**: 10 minutes

**Cook Time**: none

**Ingredients**:

- 1 ½ lbs. seedless cucumber, chopped
- 1 cup fresh chopped mint
- ¼ cup chopped green onion
- 2 cloves garlic, minced
- 1 cup canned coconut milk
- 1 tablespoon fresh lemon juice
- Salt and pepper to taste

**Instructions**:

1. Combine all of the ingredients in a blender or food processor.
2. Blend the mixture until smooth and well combined.
3. Cover and chill for 2 to 4 hours before serving.

## Creamy Mushroom Bisque

**Servings**: 4

**Prep Time**: 5 minutes

**Cook Time**: 25 minutes

**Ingredients**:

- 2 tablespoons olive oil
- 2 medium leeks, sliced (white and light green parts)
- 1 tablespoon minced garlic
- 1 lbs. sliced mushrooms
- ½ teaspoon fresh chopped thyme
- 2 cups water
- 2 cups canned coconut milk
- Salt and pepper to taste

**Instructions**:

1. Heat the oil in a stockpot over medium-high heat.
2. Add the leeks and cook for 10 minutes or so until softened.
3. Stir in the garlic, mushrooms and thyme.
4. Cook for 5 minutes, stirring.
5. Add the water and coconut milk then bring to a simmer and cook for 5 minutes.

6. Divide the soup in half and puree one half using an immersion blender.

7. Stir the blended soup into the stockpot and return to heat until heated through.

8. Season with salt and pepper to taste and serve hot.

## Carrot Ginger Soup

**Servings**: 4 to 6

**Prep Time**: 10 minutes

**Cook Time**: 25 minutes

**Ingredients**:

- 2 tablespoons olive oil
- 4 cloves garlic, minced
- 2 tablespoons fresh grated ginger
- 1 cup chopped onion
- Salt and pepper to taste
- 6 cups vegetable stock
- 2 lbs. chopped carrots
- 1 medium Yukon gold potato, chopped
- 1 teaspoon fresh chopped thyme

**Instructions**:

1. Heat the oil in stockpot over medium-high heat.
2. Add the garlic and ginger and cook for 1 minute.
3. Stir in the onion, salt and pepper and cook for 10 minutes, until the onion is tender.
4. Whisk in the vegetable stock and stir in the carrots and potato.

5. Bring the mixture to a simmer and cook, covered, for 20 minutes until the carrots are tender.

6. Remove from heat and puree the soup using an immersion blender.

7. Whisk in the coconut milk and thyme then serve hot.

## Tomato Gazpacho

**Servings**: 8

**Prep Time**: 15 minutes

**Cook Time**: none

**Ingredients**:

- 5 ripe Roma tomatoes, quartered
- 2 stalks celery, chopped
- 1 large seedless cucumber, chopped
- 1 medium zucchini, chopped
- ½ red onion, quartered
- 2 cloves garlic, peeled
- 4 cups tomato juice
- ¼ cup olive oil
- 1 tablespoon white wine vinegar
- Salt and pepper to taste

**Instructions**:

1. Place the tomatoes in a food processor and pulse until finely chopped.
2. Transfer the tomatoes to a bowl then repeat with the remaining vegetables, pulsing the garlic and red onion together last.

3. Stir together all of the vegetables in the bowl with the remaining ingredients.

4. Cover and chill for several hours before serving.

## Cream of Broccoli Soup

**Servings**: 4 to 6

**Prep Time**: 10 minutes

**Cook Time**: 15 minutes

**Ingredients**:

- 4 cups vegetable stock
- 4 stalks broccoli, chopped
- 1 tablespoon olive oil
- ½ cup diced yellow onion
- 1 teaspoon minced garlic
- 1 cup unsweetened coconut milk
- ½ teaspoon ground nutmeg
- Pinch cayenne pepper
- Salt and pepper to taste

**Instructions**:

1. Bring the broth to boil in a large saucepan over high heat.
2. Add the broccoli then simmer for 10 minutes until the broccoli is fork tender.
3. In a skillet, heat the olive oil over medium heat.

4. Add the garlic and onion and cook for 5 minutes, stirring often.
5. Stir the garlic and onion into the broccoli and broth mixture then remove from heat.
6. Puree the soup using an immersion blender then whisk in the remaining ingredients.
7. Return the soup to the heat and cook until heated through.
8. Spoon into bowls and serve hot.

## Brussels Sprouts Kale Salad

**Servings**: 2

**Prep Time**: 10 minutes

**Cook Time**: none

**Ingredients**:

- 3 cups Brussels sprouts, sliced thin
- 6 kale leaves, sliced thin
- ¼ cup raw sunflower seeds
- 3 tablespoons fresh lemon juice
- 2 tablespoons olive oil
- 1 tablespoon whole-grain mustard
- Pinch salt

**Instructions**:

1. Combine the Brussels sprouts, kale and sunflower seeds in a salad bowl.
2. Whisk together the remaining ingredients and toss with the salad to coat.
3. Chill until ready to serve.

## Colorful Cabbage Slaw

**Servings**: 4 to 6

**Prep Time**: 10 minutes

**Cook Time**: none

**Ingredients**:

- 1 small head purple cabbage, sliced thin
- 1 head romaine lettuce, chopped fine
- 2 large carrots, grated
- 2 green onions, sliced
- ½ cup tahini
- ½ cup fresh lemon juice
- 2 tablespoons olive oil
- 1 teaspoon sea salt
- Pinch dried garlic

**Instructions**:

1. Combine the cabbage, lettuce, carrots and green onion in a salad bowl.
2. Whisk together the remaining ingredients and toss with the vegetables to coat.
3. Chill until ready to serve.

## Spinach Basil Lime Salad

**Servings**: 4

**Prep Time**: 10 minutes

**Cook Time**: none

**Ingredients**:

- 8 ounces baby spinach leaves
- 1 cup fresh basil leaves
- 1 cup sliced mushroom
- 1 medium tomato, chopped
- 3 tablespoons olive oil
- 3 tablespoons fresh lime juice
- 1 teaspoon Dijon mustard
- Pinch salt and pepper
- 1 medium avocado, pitted and sliced

**Instructions**:

1. Combine the spinach, basil, mushroom and tomato in a salad bowl.
2. Whisk together the lime juice, olive oil, mustard, salt and pepper in a small bowl.
3. Toss the dressing with the salad to coat then top with sliced avocado to serve.

## Spring Fling Salad

**Servings**: 4

**Prep Time**: 10 minutes

**Cook Time**: none

**Ingredients**:

- 1 head Bibb lettuce, chopped
- 1 cup baby spinach leaves
- 1 cup fresh frisée
- 4 small radishes, sliced thin
- ¼ cup olive oil
- 1 tablespoon fresh lemon juice
- 2 teaspoons Dijon mustard
- Pinch salt and pepper

**Instructions**:

1. Combine the lettuce, spinach, frisée and radishes in a salad bowl.
2. Whisk together the remaining ingredients and toss with the salad to coat.
3. Chill until ready to serve.

## 4.) Snacks and Appetizers

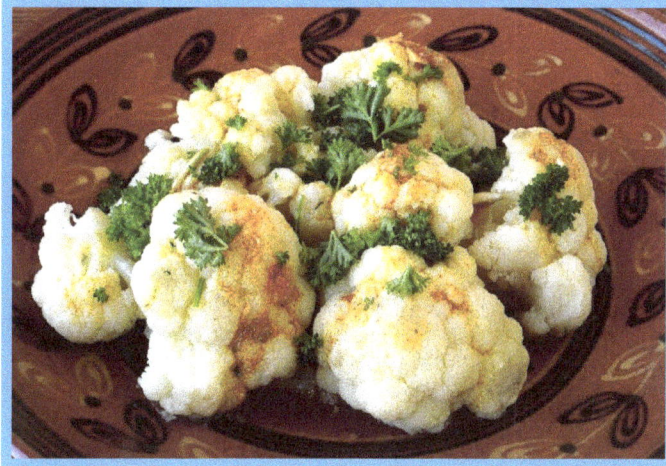

### Recipes Included in this Section:

Kale Chips

Cinnamon Applesauce

Cashew Cream with Celery

Roasted Pumpkin Seeds

Curry Roasted Cauliflower

Roast Beet Hummus

## Kale Chips

**Servings**: 4

**Prep Time**: 5 minutes

**Cook Time**:

**Ingredients**:

- 2 bunches fresh kale
- 2 tablespoons olive oil
- Coarse sea salt

**Instructions**:

1. Preheat the oven to 200°F and line a baking sheet with parchment paper.
2. Rinse the kale well then shake and pat dry.
3. Tear the kale into 2-inch chunks by hand and arrange them on the baking sheet in a single layer.
4. Drizzle the kale with olive oil and sprinkle with salt.
5. Bake for 20 minutes or until dried and crisp.

## Cinnamon Applesauce

**Servings**: 4

**Prep Time**: 5 minutes

**Cook Time**: 30 minutes

**Ingredients**:

- 3 ½ lbs. green apples, peeled and quartered
- 4 strips lemon peel
- 3 tablespoons fresh lemon juice
- 1 tablespoon ground cinnamon
- 1 cup water
- Pinch salt

**Instructions**:

1. Combine all of the ingredients in a stockpot and bring to a boil, covered.
2. Reduce heat and simmer for 20 to 30 minutes until the apples are tender.
3. Remove the lemon peel then mash the apples with a potato masher.
4. Chill until ready to serve or serve warm.

## Cashew Cream with Celery

**Servings**: 4

**Prep Time**: 5 minutes

**Cook Time**: none

**Ingredients**:

- 1 cup raw cashews
- 1 cup hot water
- 1 teaspoon ground cinnamon
- Pinch salt

**Instructions**:

1. Soak the cashews in the water for about 30 minutes.
2. Transfer the mixture to a blender along with the cinnamon and salt.
3. Blend until smooth and creamy.
4. Cover and chill until ready to serve.

## Roasted Pumpkin Seeds

**Servings**: 4 to 6

**Prep Time**: 5 minutes

**Cook Time**: 20 minutes

**Ingredients**:

- 2 cups raw pumpkin seeds, shelled
- 3 ½ tablespoons fresh lime juice
- 2 teaspoons chili powder
- 1 teaspoon coarse salt

**Instructions**:

1. Preheat the oven to 350°F and line a baking sheet with parchment paper.
2. Toss the pumpkin seeds with the lime juice, chili powder and salt.
3. Spread the seeds on the baking sheet in a single layer and bake for 10 minutes.
4. Stir the seeds then bake for another 8 to 10 minutes until browned.
5. Cool the seeds before serving.

## Curry Roasted Cauliflower

**Servings**: 4

**Prep Time**: 5 minutes

**Cook Time**: 35 minutes

**Ingredients**:

- 2 small heads cauliflower, cut into florets
- ¼ cup curry powder
- 3 tablespoons coconut oil, melted
- Salt and pepper to taste

**Instructions**:

1. Preheat the oven to 450°F.
2. Toss the cauliflower with the coconut oil, curry powder, salt and pepper.
3. Spread the cauliflower on a foil-lined baking sheet and top with another sheet of foil.
4. Bake for 15 minutes then remove the top sheet of foil and bake for 15 to 20 minutes more until lightly browned.
5. Cool the cauliflower slightly before serving.

## Roast Beet Hummus

**Servings**: 4 to 6

**Prep Time**: 10 minutes

**Cook Time**: none

**Ingredients**:

- 1 cup white cannellini beans, cooked
- ½ cup roasted beets, chopped
- ½ teaspoon minced garlic
- 2 tablespoons olive oil
- 2 tablespoons fresh lemon juice
- Pinch salt and pepper

**Instructions**:

1. Combine all of the ingredients in a food processor.
2. Blend on high speed until smooth and well blended.
3. Chill until ready to serve.
4. Serve with carrot or celery sticks for dipping.

## 5.) Main Entrees

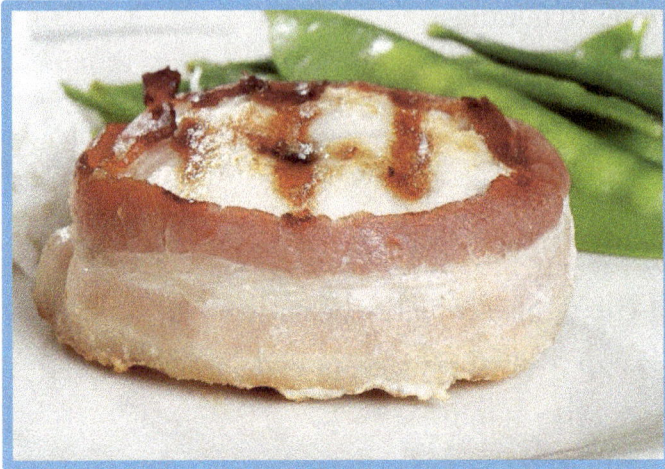

## **Recipes Included in this Section:**

Braised Lamb Shanks

Spaghetti Squash with Meat Sauce

Veggie Quinoa Burgers

Mediterranean Meatballs

Lemon Broiled Salmon

Bacon-Wrapped Chicken

Skillet Steak with Mushrooms

Cilantro Turkey Burgers

## Braised Lamb Shanks

**Servings**: 4

**Prep Time**: 15 minutes

**Cook Time**: 4 to 6 hours

**Ingredients**:

- 2 lbs. lamb shanks, boneless
- 2 tablespoons olive oil
- 4 cups marinara sauce
- 1 large yellow onion, chopped
- 1 cup sliced mushrooms
- 2 medium carrots, chopped
- 1 tablespoon minced garlic
- Salt and pepper to taste

**Instructions**:

1. Season the lamb liberally with salt and pepper to taste.
2. Heat the oil in a Dutch oven over medium-high heat then add the garlic.
3. Cook for 1 minute then add the lamb shanks.
4. Let the lamb cook for 2 to 3 minutes on each side, turning to brown evenly.

5. Add the onion, carrot and mushrooms and stir well.

6. Stir in the marinara sauce then bring to a simmer.

7. Cover and simmer the lamb for 4 to 6 hours until the lamb is falling off the bone.

## Spaghetti Squash with Meat Sauce

**Servings**: 4

**Prep Time**: 45 minutes

**Cook Time**: 45 minutes

**Ingredients**:

- 1 large spaghetti squash
- Salt and pepper to taste
- 2 tablespoons olive oil
- 1 large onion, diced
- 1 large stalk celery, diced
- 1 large carrot, diced
- 1 lbs. ground lamb
- ½ (6-ounce) can tomato paste
- ½ cup canned coconut milk

**Instructions**:

1. Preheat the oven to 375°F.
2. Cut the squash in half and scoop out the seeds.
3. Sprinkle the cut halves with salt and pepper then place them cut-side down on a baking sheet.
4. Roast the squash for 35 to 45 minutes until tender then set aside until cool enough to handle.

5. Scoop the flesh of the squash into a bowl, shredding it with a fork and set aside.
6. Heat the oil in a skillet over medium-high heat.
7. Add the onion, celery and carrots and cook for 5 to 7 minutes until tender.
8. Stir in the garlic and cook for 1 minute more.
9. Add the ground lamb and cook for 5 minutes or so until cooked through.
10. Stir in the tomato paste, coconut milk, salt and pepper and simmer over low heat for 30 minutes.
11. Serve the meat sauce hot over the spaghetti squash.

## Veggie Quinoa Burgers

**Servings**: 4

**Prep Time**: 5 minutes

**Cook Time**: 20 minutes

**Ingredients**:

2 ½ cups cooked quinoa

4 large eggs

- ½ teaspoon salt
- 1 sweet onion, diced
- 1 teaspoon minced garlic
- 1 cup almond flour
- 2 tablespoons olive oil

**Instructions**:

1. Whisk together the quinoa, eggs and salt in a mixing bowl.
2. Add the onion, garlic, almond flour and stir well.
3. Let the mixture sit for 5 minutes to absorb the moisture.
4. Shape the mixture into 1-inch patties by hand.
5. Heat the oil in a skillet over medium heat.

6. Add the patties to the hot oil then cover and cook for 7 to 10 minutes until the bottoms are evenly browned.

7. Carefully flip the patties and cook for another 7 to 10 minutes until browned.

8. Drain on paper towels and serve warm.

## Mediterranean Meatballs

**Servings**: 4

**Prep Time**: 10 minutes

**Cook Time**: 25 minutes

**Ingredients**:

- 1 lbs. ground lamb
- 1 teaspoon minced garlic
- 2 tablespoons minced onion
- 1 tablespoon olive oil
- 1 teaspoon lemon zest
- ½ teaspoon dried oregano
- ½ teaspoon sea salt
- ¼ teaspoon garlic powder
- Pepper to taste

**Instructions**:

1. Preheat the oven to 400°F and line a baking sheet with foil.
2. Combine all of the ingredients in a mixing bowl and stir well.
3. Shape the mixture by hand into 1 ½ inch balls.

4. Arrange the balls on the baking sheet and bake for 20 to 25 minutes until cooked through.

## Lemon Broiled Salmon

**Servings**: 4

**Prep Time**: 5 minutes

**Cook Time**: 15 minutes

**Ingredients**:

- 4 (4 to 6-ounce) salmon fillets
- 2 tablespoons coconut oil
- 1 to 2 tablespoons lemon zest
- Salt and pepper to taste
- 1 lemon, sliced thin

**Instructions**:

1. Preheat the broiler in your oven to the low heat setting.
2. Grease the bottom of a baking dish with coconut oil.
3. Season the salmon fillets with salt and pepper to taste and place them in the baking dish.
4. Sprinkle the salmon with lemon zest and top each fillet with a slice or two of lemon.
5. Broil for 10 to 15 minutes or until cooked to the desired temperature.

## Bacon-Wrapped Chicken

**Servings**: 4

**Prep Time**: 5 minutes

**Cook Time**: 40 minutes

**Ingredients**:

- 4 boneless chicken thighs
- 1 teaspoon chili powder
- ½ teaspoon garlic powder
- Pinch cayenne pepper
- Salt and pepper to taste
- 8 slices uncooked bacon

**Instructions**:

1. Preheat the oven to 375°F.
2. Combine the chili powder, garlic powder, cayenne, salt and pepper in a small bowl.
3. Season the chicken thighs with the spice mix then wrap each in two slices of bacon.
4. Place the chicken thighs in a baking dish and sprinkle any remaining spice mixture on top.
5. Bake for 40 minutes or until the chicken is cooked through.

## Skillet Steak with Mushrooms

**Servings**: 4

**Prep Time**: 10 minutes

**Cook Time**: 15 minutes

**Ingredients**:

- ½ lbs. skillet steak
- 1 medium onion, sliced
- 8 oz. sliced mushrooms
- 1 tablespoon plus 1 teaspoon olive oil
- Salt and pepper to taste

**Instructions**:

1. Carefully slice the steak into thin strips and season with salt and pepper to taste.
2. Heat ½ tablespoon oil in a large skillet over high heat.
3. Add the strips of steak and cook for 1 minute then turn and cook for another 30 to 45 seconds until just browned.
4. Transfer the beef to a bowl and set aside.
5. Add another ½ tablespoon oil along with the onions to the skillet and season with salt and pepper.

6. Cook for 2 to 3 minutes until the onions are just browned.

7. Add the remaining olive oil to the skillet and stir in the mushrooms.

8. Cook for 3 minutes, stirring once or twice.

9. Add the steak back to the skillet, stirring until just heated through. Serve hot.

## Cilantro Turkey Burgers

**Servings**: 4

**Prep Time**: 5 minutes

**Cook Time**: 15 minutes

**Ingredients**:

- 1 lbs. lean ground turkey
- 1 teaspoon minced garlic
- 2 tablespoons minced red onion
- ¼ cup chopped cilantro
- 1 teaspoon dried parsley
- Salt and pepper to taste

**Instructions**:

1. Preheat the broiler in your oven to high heat.
2. Combine all of the ingredients in a mixing bowl and stir well.
3. Shape the mixture into four even-sized patties by hand, patting them to about ½-inch thick.
4. Arrange the patties on a broiler pan and broil for 5 to 7 minutes on each side until cooked through.
5. Serve hot on a bed of lettuce with your favorite burger toppings.

## 6.) Side Dishes

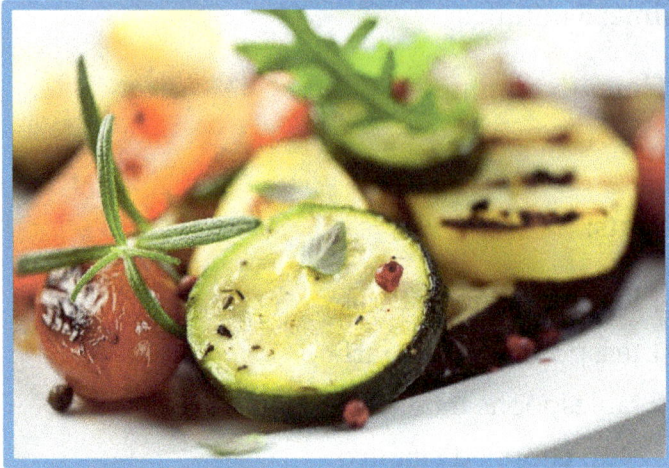

### Recipes Included in this Section:

Roasted Beets

Lemon Sautéed Collard Greens

Rosemary Roasted Veggies

Mashed Cauliflower

Green Bean Casserole

## Roasted Beets

**Servings**: 4

**Prep Time**: 5 minutes

**Cook Time**: 1 ½ hours

**Ingredients**:

- 4 medium beets
- 1 tablespoon olive oil
- Salt and pepper to taste

**Instructions**:

1. Preheat the oven to 375°F.
2. Rinse the beats well, scrubbing them if needed.
3. Wrap the beats up in a piece of foil and place on the center rack.
4. Roast the beets for 1 to 1 ½ hours until tender then remove from the oven to cool slightly.
5. Remove the beets from the aluminum foil and slice or chop.
6. Toss the beets with olive oil, salt and pepper to serve.

## Lemon Sautéed Collard Greens

**Servings**: 4

**Prep Time**: 10 minutes

**Cook Time**: 15 minutes

**Ingredients**:

- 2 bunches fresh collard greens
- 1 tablespoon olive oil
- 1 tablespoon minced garlic
- 1 tablespoon fresh lemon juice
- 1 teaspoon lemon zest

**Instructions**:

1. Rinse the collard greens well and shake dry.
2. Trim the stems and ribs from the collard greens and chop into 1-inch pieces.
3. Bring a pot of water to boil and add the collard greens – boil for 10 minutes then drain.
4. Heat the oil in a skillet over medium-high heat.
5. Add the garlic and cook for 1 minute.
6. Stir in the cooked collard greens and cook for 5 minutes, stirring well.

7. Drizzle with lemon juice and stir in the lemon zest to serve.

## Rosemary Roasted Veggies

**Servings**: 4 to 6

**Prep Time**: 5 minutes

**Cook Time**: 45 minutes

**Ingredients**:

- 2 cups chopped broccoli florets
- 2 cups chopped cauliflower florets
- 1 cup baby carrots
- 1 medium zucchini, cut into 1-inch chunks
- 1 sweet yellow onion, quartered
- 3 tablespoons olive oil
- 2 tablespoons dried rosemary
- ¼ cup vegetable stock

**Instructions**:

1. Preheat the oven to 400°F.
2. Combine the broccoli, cauliflower, carrot, onion and zucchini in a large bowl.
3. Toss with the olive oil and rosemary then transfer to a glass baking dish, spreading evenly.
4. Drizzle with vegetable stock then roast for 25 minutes.

5. Turn the vegetables then roast for another 20 minutes or so until tender.

## Mashed Cauliflower

**Servings**: 4

**Prep Time**: 5 minutes

**Cook Time**: 10 minutes

**Ingredients**:

- 1 large head cauliflower, chopped
- 2 tablespoons roasted garlic
- 1 tablespoon fresh chopped chives
- Salt and pepper to taste

**Instructions**:

1. Place a steamer insert in a large saucepan and fill the pan with 1 inch of water.
2. Bring the water to a boil then add the cauliflower.
3. Simmer, covered, for 6 to 8 minutes until the cauliflower is tender.
4. Drain the cauliflower then transfer to a large bowl.
5. Mash the cauliflower with a potato masher then stir in the remaining ingredients.

## Green Bean Casserole

**Servings**: 6

**Prep Time**: 45 minutes

**Cook Time**: 30 minutes

**Ingredients**:

- 2 tablespoons olive oil
- 1 large yellow onion, sliced thin
- 2 cups chopped parsnips
- 10 ounces sliced mushrooms
- 1 tablespoon minced garlic
- 1 ½ cups water
- 1 ½ teaspoons salt
- 1 lbs. green beans, trimmed

**Instructions**:

1. Heat half the oil in a skillet over medium heat.
2. Add the onion and sauté for 25 minutes or so until caramelized.
3. Transfer the onions to a bowl and set aside.
4. Reheat the skillet and sauté the mushrooms and garlic until browned – about 5 minutes. Set aside.

5. Place a steamer basket in a large saucepan and fill the pan with 1 inch of water.

6. Add the chopped parsnips then bring the water to a boil.

7. Cover and simmer for 8 minutes until the parsnips are tender.

8. Drain the parsnips and transfer to a food processor to cool.

9. Steam the beans for 6 to 8 minutes using the same process then drain them and place them in a glass baking dish.

10. Top the green beans with half the mushrooms then place the rest in the blender.

11. Blend the parsnips and mushrooms with 1 ½ cups water and 1 ½ teaspoons salt until creamy.

12. Pour the mixture over the green beans and top with caramelized onions.

13. Bake for 30 minutes at 350°F until hot and bubbling.

## 7.) Desserts

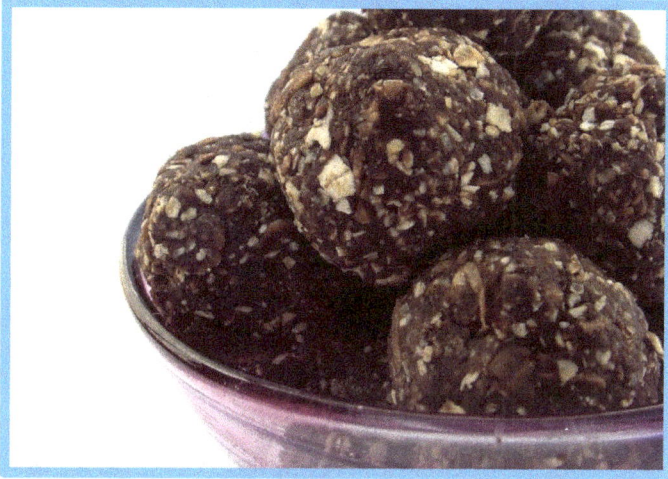

### Recipes Included in this Section:

Raw Cocoa Date Truffles

Pumpkin Mug Cake

Carrot Cake Pudding

Stuffed Apples

Pumpkin Chocolate Fudge

Lemon Chia Pudding

Choco-Coconut Almond Balls

Avocado Chocolate Mousse

## Cocoa Date Truffles

**Servings**: 4

**Prep Time**: 10 minutes

**Cook Time**: none

**Ingredients**:

- ½ cup raw sunflower seeds
- ½ cup raw cashews
- ½ cup pitted Medjool dates
- 3 to 4 tablespoons unsweetened cocoa powder
- Pinch salt

**Instructions**:

1. Combine the sunflower seeds and cashews in a food processor and blend until finely chopped.
2. Add the remaining ingredients and blend until it forms a sticky mixture.
3. Roll the mixture into 1-inch balls by hand and place them on a tray or plate.
4. Chill the truffles until firm.

## Pumpkin Mug Cake

**Servings**: 1

**Prep Time**: 3 minutes

**Cook Time**: 3 minutes

**Ingredients**:

- 2 tablespoons canned coconut milk
- 1 ½ tablespoons coconut flour
- 1 tablespoon pumpkin puree
- 1 tablespoon ghee
- 1 teaspoon vanilla extract
- ½ teaspoon pumpkin pie spice
- ¼ teaspoon baking soda
- Pinch salt

**Instructions**:

1. Whisk together all of the ingredients in a greased microwave-safe mug until smooth.
2. Microwave on high heat for 1 ½ to 2 ½ minutes until cooked through.
3. Let the cake cool for 2 to 3 minutes before serving.

## Carrot Cake Pudding

**Servings**: 4

**Prep Time**: 5 minutes

**Cook Time**: 25 minutes

**Ingredients**:

- 2 cups chopped carrots
- 2 tablespoons coconut butter
- 2 tablespoons almond butter
- 1 teaspoon vanilla extract
- ¾ teaspoon ground cinnamon
- Pinch ground nutmeg
- Pinch sea salt

**Instructions**:

1. Place the carrots in medium saucepan and cover with water.
2. Bring the carrots to a simmer over medium heat and cook for 20 to 25 minutes until soft.
3. Drain the carrots and transfer them to a food processor.
4. Blend the carrots until pureed then add the rest of the ingredients to the food processor.

5.  Blend until smooth then spoon into bowls to serve.

## Stuffed Apples

**Servings**: 4

**Prep Time**: 10 minutes

**Cook Time**: 2 to 3 hours

**Ingredients**:

- 4 green apples
- ½ cup melted coconut butter
- ¼ cup almond butter
- 1 ½ tablespoons ground cinnamon
- ¼ teaspoon ground nutmeg
- Pinch sea salt
- ¼ cup unsweetened shredded coconut

**Instructions**:

1. Core the apples and place them upright inside your slow cooker.
2. Whisk together the coconut butter and almond butter until smooth.
3. Blend in the cinnamon, nutmeg and salt then spoon the mixture into the cored apples.
4. Sprinkle the apples with shredded coconut and cover the slow cooker.

5. Cook on low heat for 2 to 3 hours until the apples are tender.

## Pumpkin Chocolate Fudge

**Servings**: 10 to 12

**Prep Time**: 5 minutes

**Cook Time**: none

**Ingredients**:

- 1 cup melted coconut butter
- 1 cup pumpkin puree
- ½ cup almond butter
- ¼ cup raw cocoa powder
- 3 tablespoons melted coconut oil
- 1 teaspoon vanilla extract
- Pinch ground cinnamon

**Instructions**:

1. Combine all of the ingredients in a food processor and blend until smooth.
2. Line a square or rectangular baking dish with parchment and spread the fudge evenly inside it.
3. Cover and chill for 4 hours then cut the fudge into squares to enjoy.

## Lemon Chia Pudding

**Servings**: 4

**Prep Time**: 5 minutes

**Cook Time**: none

**Ingredients**:

- 1 (12 ounce) can full-fat coconut milk
- ¼ cup raw chia seeds
- 2 tablespoons fresh lemon juice
- ¼ teaspoon fresh lemon zest

**Instructions**:

1. Whisk together all of the ingredients in a bowl until well combined.
2. Cover and chill in the refrigerator for at least 2 hours until set.
3. Spoon into bowls to serve.

## Choco-Coconut Almond Balls

**Servings**: 8 to 10

**Prep Time**: 10 minutes

**Cook Time**: none

**Ingredients**:

- ¾ cup almond butter
- ¼ cup plus 1 tablespoon unsweetened coconut
- 2 ½ teaspoons unsweetened cocoa powder
- 1 teaspoon vanilla extract
- Pinch ground cinnamon

**Instructions**:

1. Whisk together all ingredients in a mixing bowl until smooth.
2. Shape the mixture into 1-inch balls by hand and arrange them on a parchment-lined baking sheet.
3. Chill the balls in the freezer for 10 to 15 minutes until firm.
4. Store in the freezer until ready to enjoy.

## Avocado Chocolate Mousse

**Servings**: 2

**Prep Time**: 10 minutes

**Cook Time**: none

**Ingredients**:

- 2 ripe avocados, pitted
- 2 under-ripe bananas, peeled
- ½ cup unsweetened coconut milk
- ½ cup unsweetened cocoa powder
- ¾ teaspoon vanilla extract
- Pinch ground cinnamon

**Instructions**:

1. Place the avocado in a food processor with the banana and blend until smooth.
2. Add the remaining ingredients and blend for 30 seconds on high speed or until creamy.
3. Spoon the mousse into dishes and chill until ready to serve.

# Chapter Six: Sugar Detox Meal Plan

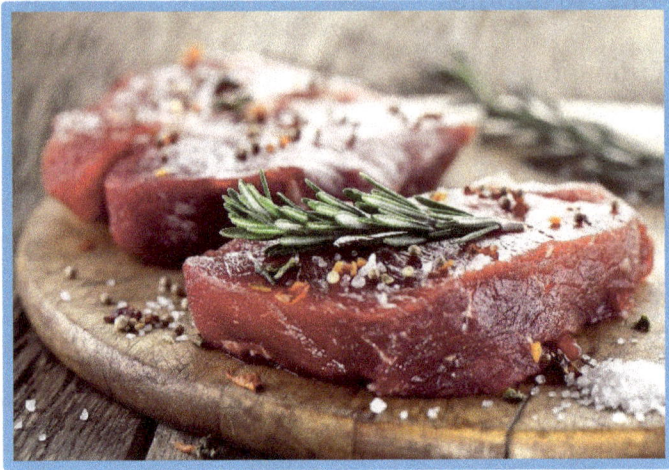

The recipes from the previous chapter are your secret to success in the sugar detox – without a repertoire of recipes to draw from, you are likely to get into a rut and go off the diet. If you are serious about following the sugar detox all the way through, you would be wise to not only use these recipes but to create a plan for your detox. Planning your meals ensures that you don't have to waste time figuring out what you are going to eat – it also means that you make the most of your shopping trips. In this chapter you will find a 30-day detox meal plan to guide you through the process using recipes from this book.

## 1.) Sugar Detox Week 1

### Day One:

Breakfast – Pumpkin Cinnamon Pancakes

Lunch – Cool Cucumber Soup

Dinner – Braised Lamb Shanks

Snack/Dessert – Kale Chips

### Day Two:

Breakfast – Super Green Mint Smoothie

Lunch – Brussels Sprouts Kale Salad

Dinner – Spaghetti Squash with Meat Sauce

Snack/Dessert – Raw Cocoa Date Truffles

### Day Three:

Breakfast – Single-Serve Egg Cups

Lunch – Creamy Mushroom Bisque

Dinner – Veggie Quinoa Burgers

Snack/Dessert – Cinnamon Applesauce

## Day Four:

Breakfast – Spicy Carrot Tomato Juice

Lunch – Colorful Cabbage Slaw

Dinner – Mediterranean Meatballs

Snack/Dessert – Roasted Beets

## Day Five:

Breakfast – Carrot Pumpkin Muffins

Lunch – Carrot Ginger Soup

Dinner – Lemon Broiled Salmon

Snack/Dessert – Carrot Cake Pudding

## Day Six:

Breakfast – Avocado Cucumber Smoothie

Lunch – Spinach Basil Lime Salad

Dinner – Bacon-Wrapped Chicken

Snack/Dessert – Cashew Cream with Celery

## Day Seven:

Breakfast – Walnut Breakfast Quinoa

Lunch – Tomato Gazpacho

Dinner – Skillet Steak with Mushrooms

Snack/Dessert – Pumpkin Mug Cake

## 2.) Sugar Detox Week 2

### Day One:

Breakfast – Fresh Celery Kale Juice

Lunch – Spring Fling Salad

Dinner – Cilantro Turkey Burgers

Snack/Dessert – Curry Roasted Cauliflower

### Day Two:

Breakfast – Coconut Flour Pancakes

Lunch – Cream of Broccoli Soup

Dinner – Braised Lamb Shanks

Snack/Dessert – Stuffed Apples

### Day Three:

Breakfast – Tomato Basil Omelet

Lunch – Colorful Cabbage Slaw

Dinner – Spaghetti Squash with Meat Sauce

Snack/Dessert – Lemon Chia Pudding

## Day Four:

Breakfast – Refreshing Cilantro Lime Smoothie

Lunch – Creamy Mushroom Bisque

Dinner – Veggie Quinoa Burgers

Snack/Dessert – Roasted Beet Hummus

## Day Five:

Breakfast – Almond Flour Muffins

Lunch – Brussels Sprouts Kale Salad

Dinner – Mediterranean Meatballs

Snack/Dessert – Rosemary Roasted Veggies

## Day Six:

Breakfast – Simple Salad Greens Juice

Lunch – Spinach Basil Lime Salad

Dinner – Lemon Broiled Salmon

Snack/Dessert – Pumpkin Chocolate Fudge

## Day Seven:

Breakfast – Buckwheat Porridge

Lunch – Cool Cucumber Soup

Dinner – Bacon-Wrapped Chicken

Snack/Dessert – Roasted Pumpkin Seeds

### 3.) Sugar Detox Week 3

## Day One:

Breakfast – Broccoli Beet Smoothie

Lunch – Spring Fling Salad

Dinner – Carrot Ginger Soup

Snack/Dessert – Choco-Coconut Almond Balls

## Day Two:

Breakfast – Mushroom Scallion Omelet

Lunch – Tomato Gazpacho

Dinner – Skillet Steak with Mushrooms

Snack/Dessert – Cinnamon Applesauce

## Day Three:

Breakfast – Parsley Mint Juice with Lime

Lunch – Colorful Cabbage Slaw

Dinner – Cream of Broccoli Soup

Snack/Dessert – Carrot Cake Pudding

## Day Four:

Breakfast – Cinnamon Baked Quinoa

Lunch – Brussels Sprouts and Kale Salad

Dinner – Cilantro Turkey Burgers

Snack/Dessert – Kale Chips

## Day Five:

Breakfast – Almond Spinach Smoothie

Lunch – Creamy Mushroom Bisque

Dinner – Veggie Quinoa Burgers

Snack/Dessert – Avocado Chocolate Mousse

## Day Six:

Breakfast – Carrot Pumpkin Muffins

Lunch – Spinach Basil Lime Salad

Dinner – Braised Lamb Shanks

Snack/Dessert – Cashew Cream with Celery

## Day Seven:

Breakfast – Ginger Beet Juice

Lunch – Carrot Ginger Soup

Dinner – Mediterranean Meatballs

Snack/Dessert – Pumpkin Mug Cake

## 4.) Sugar Detox Week 4

## Day One:

Breakfast – Coconut Flour Pancakes

Lunch – Tomato Gazpacho

Dinner – Spaghetti Squash with Meat Sauce

Snack/Dessert – Raw Cocoa Date Truffles

## Day Two:

Breakfast – Avocado Cucumber Smoothie

Lunch – Creamy Mushroom Bisque

Dinner – Lemon Broiled Salmon

Snack/Dessert – Roasted Beet Hummus

## Day Three:

Breakfast – Tomato Basil Omelet

Lunch – Colorful Cabbage Slaw

Dinner – Bacon-Wrapped Chicken

Snack/Dessert – Stuffed Apples

## Day Four:

Breakfast – Fresh Celery Kale Juice

Lunch – Cool Cucumber Soup

Dinner – Skillet Steak with Mushrooms

Snack/Dessert – Curry Roasted Cauliflower

## Day Five:

Breakfast – Walnut Breakfast Quinoa

Lunch – Spinach Basil Lime Salad

Dinner – Cilantro Turkey Burgers

Snack/Dessert – Lemon Chia Pudding

## Day Six:

Breakfast – Super Green Mint Smoothie

Lunch – Spring Fling Salad

Dinner – Braised Lamb Shanks

Snack/Dessert – Roasted Pumpkin Seeds

**Day Seven:**

Breakfast – Almond Flour Muffins

Lunch – Cream of Broccoli Soup

Dinner – Veggie Quinoa Burgers

Snack/Dessert – Pumpkin Chocolate Fudge

# Chapter Seven: Relevant Websites

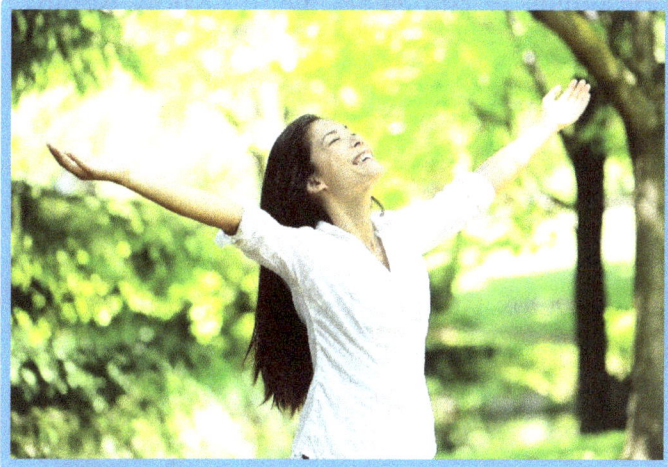

Within the pages of this book, you will find all the information you need to prepare for and to get started on a sugar detox. If you truly want to succeed in meeting your goals, you would be wise to learn everything you can about detoxing – that is where this chapter comes into play. In this chapter you will find valuable resources for detoxing tips, information about sugar addiction and additional sugar detox recipes. If you want to learn more about detoxing your body, look no further than the next few pages!

## 1.) Tips for Detoxing

Beljanski, Sylvie. "9 Things You Didn't Know About Detoxing." Marie Claire. <http://www.marieclaire.com/health-fitness/advice/at-home-detoxing-detox-facts>

"Total Body Detox Tips and Tricks." Natural Health Techniques. <http://naturalhealthtechniques.com/specificdiseasesdetoxification.htm>

"21-Day Sugar Detox." Wellness with Rose. <http://www.rosecole.com/handouts/21DaySugarDetox.pdf >

"Favorite Detox Tips." Natural Health – For a Balanced, Blissful Life. <http://www.naturalhealthmag.com/health/detox-tips>

"Daily Detoxing Tips." Whole Living – Body and Soul in Balance. <http://www.wholeliving.com/133627/daily-detoxing-tips>

## 2.) Dangers of Sugar Addiction

"Slideshow: The Truth About Sugar Addiction." WebMD.
<http://www.webmd.com/diet/ss/slideshow-sugar-addiction>

Barclay, Eliza. "Is Sugar Addiction Why So Many January Diets Fail?" NPR.org.
<http://www.npr.org/blogs/thesalt/2014/01/08/260781785/is-sugar-addiction-why-so-many-january-diets-fail>

Hyman, Mark. "Stopping Sugar Addiction: Willpower or Genetics?" The Daniel Plan.
<http://danielplan.com/healthyhabits/sugaraddiction/>

Pagoto, Sherry. "How to Get Over Your Sugar Addiction." Psychology Today.
<http://www.psychologytoday.com/blog/shrink/201209/how-get-over-your-sugar-addiction>

## 3.) Sugar Detox Recipes

"Articles, Recipes and Podcasts." 21-Day Sugar Detox, Balanced Bites. <http://balancedbites.com/the-21-day-sugar-detox-articles-recipes-podcasts>

"9 Delicious Vegan and Gluten-Free Detox Recipes." Oh She Glows. <http://ohsheglows.com/2013/12/29/9-delicious-vegan-and-gluten-free-detox-recipes/>

"25 Delicious and Clean Detox Dishes." Prevention. <http://www.prevention.com/mind-body/natural-remedies/25-delicious-and-clean-detox-dishes>

"Easy-to-Make Recipes to Detox the Year Away." FitSugar. <http://www.fitsugar.com/Healthy-Detox-Recipes-26314372#photo-10>

"Chef 21 Day Sugar Detox." Fast Paleo -- Share the Hunger. <http://fastpaleo.com/author/balancedbites/>

# Index

## A

| | |
|---|---|
| addiction | 9, 10, 13, 123, 125,133, 134 |
| antioxidants | 6 |

## B

| | |
|---|---|
| beauty products | 5, 8 |
| benefit | 2, 4, 10, 15, 24, 25 |
| benefits | 10, 11, 23 |
| blender | 16, 27, 28, 29, 30, 31, 56, 58, 60, 64, 72, 98 |
| breakfast | 3, 16, 37, 51, 111, 112, 113, 114, 115, 116, 117, 118, 119, 120, 121, 122 |

## C

| | |
|---|---|
| chemicals | 5 |
| clean eating | 5 |
| colon | 6, 8 |
| colon cleanse | 8 |
| craving | 2, 9, 10, 21, 133 |

## D

| | |
|---|---|
| dehydrator | 17 |
| desserts | 3, 99, 111, 112, 113, 114, 115, 116, 117, 118, 119, 120, 121, 122 |
| detoxification | 5, 6, 8, 23, 124 |

## V

## W

# References

"5 Benefits of a Detox Cleanse." Medical Meals. <http://blog.mymedicalmeals.com/detox/detox-cleanse-health-benefits/>

"21-Day Sugar Detox." Wellness with Rose. <http://www.rosecole.com/handouts/21DaySugarDetox.pdf>

"Articles, Recipes and Podcasts." 21-Day Sugar Detox, Balanced Bites. <http://balancedbites.com/the-21-day-sugar-detox-articles-recipes-podcasts>

"Body Systems." Detox Blog. <http://whydetox.net/body-systems>

"Detox Diets: Cleansing the Body." WebMD. <http://www.webmd.com/diet/features/detox-diets-cleansing-body?page=3>

"Detox Fitness Plan." Whole Living.
<http://www.wholeliving.com/135925/detox-fitness-plan/@center/144798/whole-body-action-plan>


"Expert Answers on Digesting Protein, Exercising During a Detox and More." Experience Life.
<http://experiencelife.com/article/expert-answers-on-digesting-protein-exercising-during-a-detox-and-more/>


Layne, Amy. "The Sugar Detox – Kiss Your Sugar Cravings Goodbye." DAMY Health.
<http://www.damyhealth.com/2011/02/the-sugar-detox/>


Pagoto, Sherry. "How to Get Over Your Sugar Addiction." Psychology Today.
<http://www.psychologytoday.com/blog/shrink/201209/how-get-over-your-sugar-addiction>


"The 21-Day Sugar Detox." Balanced Bites by Diane Sanfilippo. <http://balancedbites.com/sugar-addiction-detox>

"The Truth About Sugar Addiction." WebMD.
<http://www.webmd.com/diet/ss/slideshow-sugar-
addiction>


"Top 10 Most Common Environmental Toxins."
Canada.com. <http://www.canada.com/vancouversun/
news/story.html?id=57586947-9466-4fcf-bb1b-
2c464dd19e5c>

# Photo Credits

All photos used in this book were purchased from BigStockPhoto.com and are licensed for commercial use.

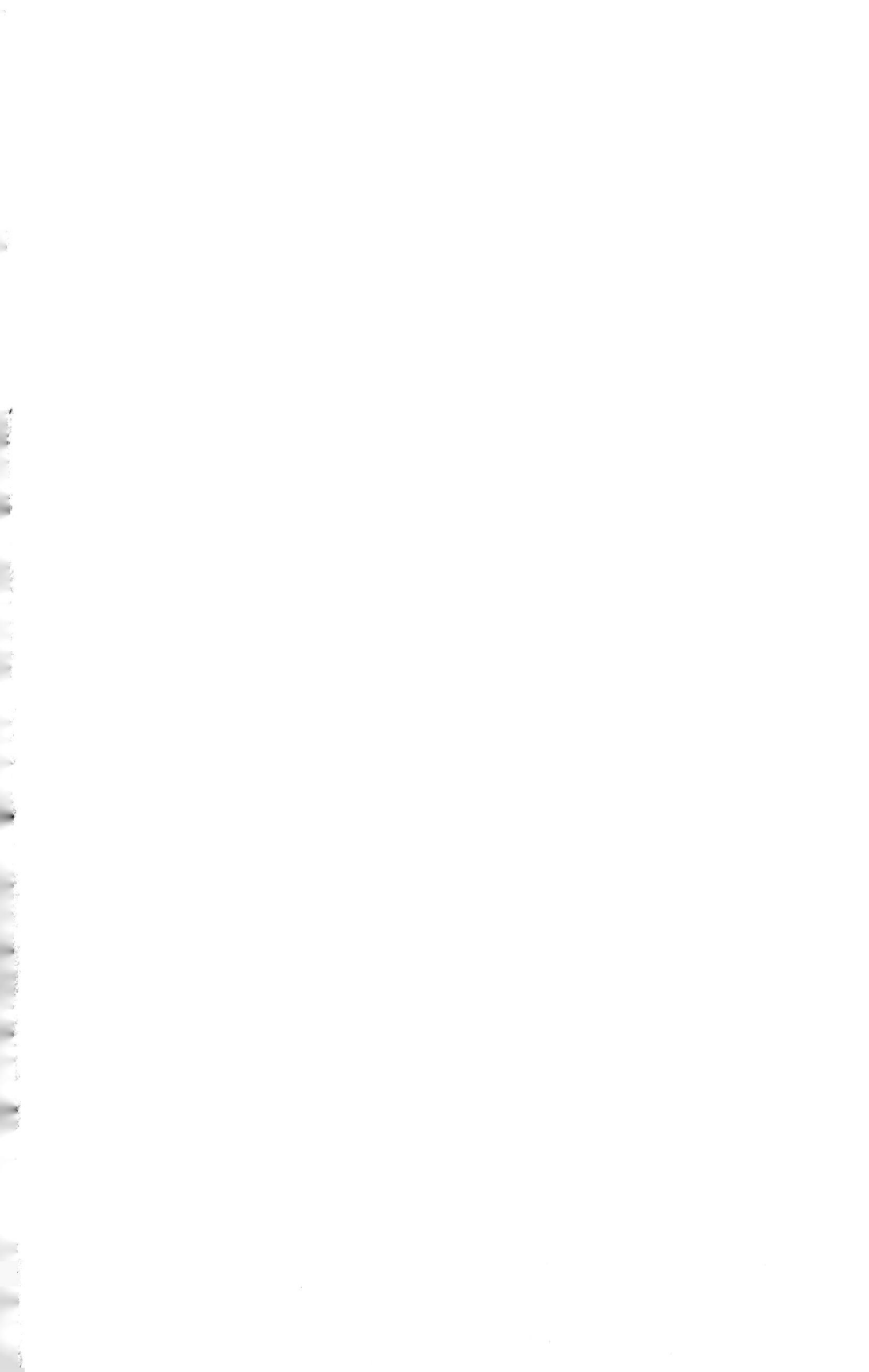

www.ingramcontent.com/pod-product-compliance
Lightning Source LLC
Chambersburg PA
CBHW060904280326
41934CB00007B/1183